Mini Materia Medica

Dr Víctor Denis Purcell

Published by Dr Víctor Denis Purcell, 2024.

MINI MATERIA MEDICA

First edition. February 6, 2024.

ISBN: 979-8224171781

Written by Dr Víctor Denis Purcell.

Mini Materia Medica

Disclaimer: The content provided herein is for entertainment purposes only and is not intended as medical advice. The information and discussions are not a substitute for professional medical opinions, diagnosis, or treatment. Always seek the advice of your physician or other qualified health provider with any questions you may have regarding a medical condition. Never disregard professional medical advice or delay seeking it because of something you have read or seen in this content.

This following presentation is a selection of the most frequent homeopathic remedies used that would be a very welcome adjunct to your home or travel medical kit.

Harmonizing Health: The Essence of Homeopathic Healing

Embarking on a journey through the world of homeopathy reveals a treasure trove of natural remedies, each with unique healing properties and applications. Among this rich assortment, specific remedies stand out for their versatility and efficacy in addressing everyday ailments, offering gentle yet powerful solutions to common health challenges. Rooted in the principle of "like cures like," these remedies work harmoniously with the body's natural healing mechanisms, gently nudging it towards balance and well-being.

Whether it's the fortifying touch of Calc Phos for growth and recovery, the soothing embrace of Calendula for skin and wound healing, or the swift action of Cantharis against painful irritations, these remedies encapsulate the essence of homeopathy's holistic approach to health. As we delve deeper into the profiles and applications of these esteemed remedies, we uncover the art and science of homeopathy, where each remedy is meticulously prepared and prescribed to resonate with the individual's unique constellation of symptoms and constitution. This personalized approach ensures that the chosen remedy aligns perfectly with the person's needs, offering a tailored path to healing and vitality.

In everyday health care, the accessibility and safety of these remedies make them invaluable allies. From the minor bumps and bruises of daily life to more persistent health concerns, they provide a compassionate and effective healing touch, embodying the gentle power of nature in every dose.

Homeopathy: A Personalized Approach to Wellness

Homeopathy's strength lies in its individualized treatment, recognizing that each person's experience of illness is unique. This segment delves into the holistic assessment process, emphasizing the importance of understanding the patient's physical, emotional, and mental state to select the most appropriate remedy.

Safety and Accessibility: The Homeopathic Advantage

The Mini Materia Medica presentation reassures the audience of the non-toxic nature of homeopathic remedies and their suitability for all ages. It also touches on the global availability and affordability of these remedies, making homeopathy a widely accessible form of healthcare.

Integrating Homeopathy into Daily Life

These homeopathic remedies deal with everyday health issues and provide, tips on building a basic homeopathic kit for common ailments like bruises, colds, and digestive upsets. The goal is to empower individuals to participate in their health and well-being actively.

Conclusion: Embracing Natural Healing

This pamphlet focuses on the benefits of integrating homeopathy into one's healthcare regimen, emphasizing its role in promoting natural, gentle healing and maintaining balance within the body. It invites the audience to explore homeopathy as a complement to conventional medicine, fostering a holistic approach to health and wellness.

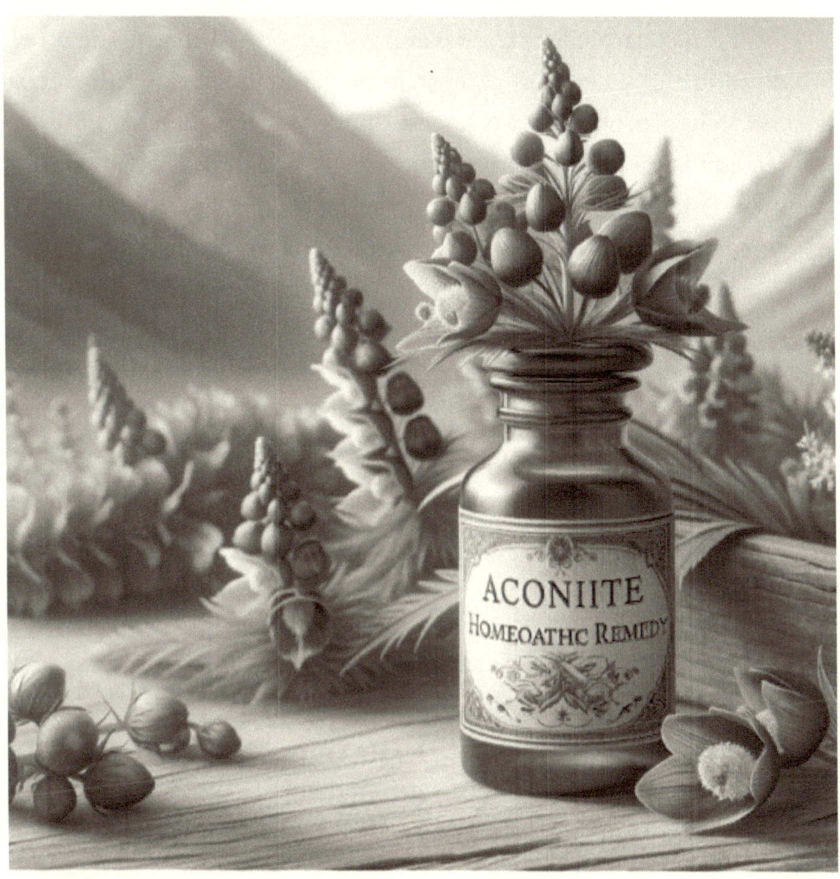

Aconite:

Introduction: Aconite, derived from the plant Aconitum napellus, also known as monkshood or wolfsbane, is a foundational homeopathic remedy recognized for its efficacy in treating sudden, acute conditions often arising from shock, fear, or exposure to cold winds. It is particularly noted for its rapid action in cases of high fever, acute inflammation, and the initial stages of respiratory infections, where symptoms develop suddenly and with intensity.

Homeopathic Preparation and Application: Through the process of dilution and succussion, Aconite is prepared in a manner that enhances its healing properties while ensuring safety for therapeutic use. This remedy is most commonly indicated for the very onset of conditions such as fever, fright, shock, and the early stages of colds and coughs, where there is a sudden and intense onset of symptoms.

Mental Symptoms: Aconite addresses a variety of mental and cognitive symptoms, including:

• Acute Fear: Intense, sudden fear, often with a fear of death, that may arise after a shock or fright.

• Restlessness: Extreme restlessness and anxiety, feeling agitated and unable to stay still.

• Panic Attacks: Sudden onset of panic attacks, with palpitations and a fear of impending doom.

Emotional Symptoms: The emotional profile for Aconite includes:

• Agitation: Emotional agitation and distress, particularly in response to sudden events or shocks.

• Sensitivity to Stimuli: Increased sensitivity to environmental stimuli, becoming easily startled or frightened.

• Impatience: A sense of urgency and impatience, wanting immediate relief or action.

Psychological Symptoms: Psychologically, Aconite is suited for:

• Shock from Traumatic Events: Psychological shock following a traumatic or frightening event, leading to acute stress symptoms.

• Overwhelming Feelings of being overwhelmed by the intensity of sudden symptoms or emotional experiences.

• Hyper-alertness: A state of hyper-alertness where the individual is jumpy and on edge, especially after a fright.

Physical Symptoms: Aconite is particularly effective in treating physical symptoms such as:

• Sudden High Fever: Rapid onset of high fever with dry, hot skin and often absent sweating.

• Acute Inflammation: Inflammatory conditions that arise suddenly, such as acute conjunctivitis or sore throat, with a sensation of burning and dryness.

• Early Stages of Colds: The initial stages of colds, particularly after exposure to cold, dry wind, with sneezing and dry nasal passages.

• Respiratory Distress: Sudden onset of respiratory symptoms like croup or asthma, especially after exposure to cold.

• Palpitations: Heart palpitations and tightness in the chest arising from acute fear or anxiety.

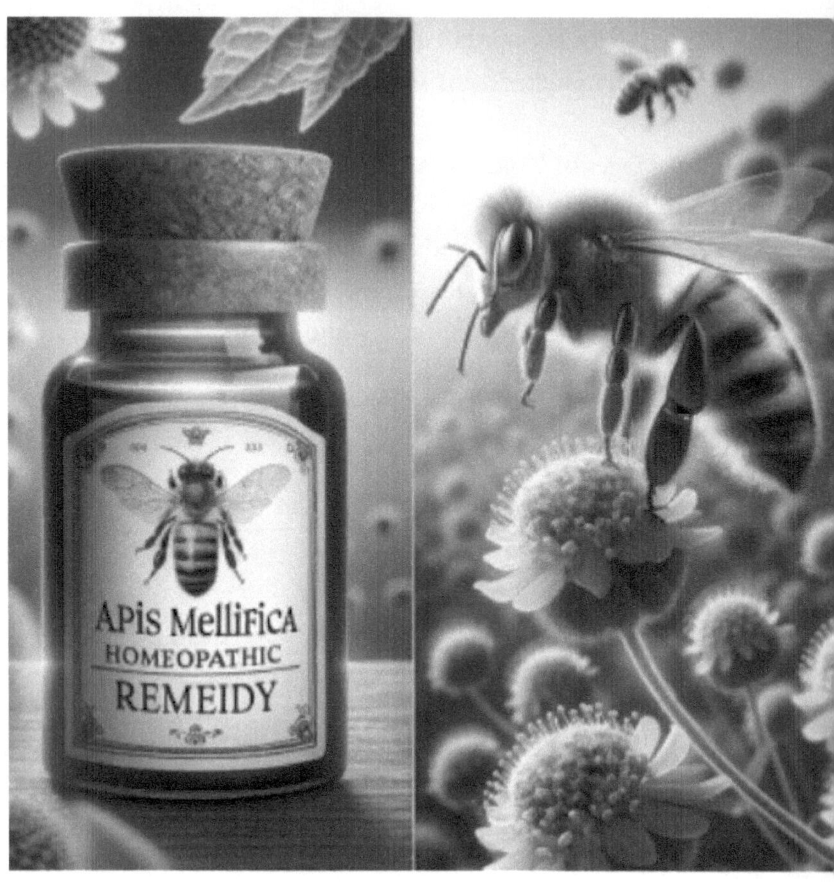

Apis Mellifica:

Introduction: Apis Mellifica, commonly known as Apis, is a prominent homeopathic remedy derived from the honeybee. It plays a significant role in homeopathy for its effectiveness in treating conditions characterized by swelling, redness, and stinging pain, mirroring the effects of a bee sting. Apis is particularly revered for its application in acute inflammatory conditions, edema, and allergic reactions.

Homeopathic Preparation and Application: Following homeopathic traditions, Apis Mellifica is meticulously prepared through dilution and succussion, which is believed to enhance its healing properties while eliminating the toxic effects of bee venom. It is predominantly utilized to address issues such as skin inflammations, urticaria, acute sore throat, and various forms of edema, significantly when symptoms improve with cold applications.

Mental Symptoms: Apis Mellifica is noted for its influence on the mental and emotional states, characterized by:

- Jealousy: A notable feature is the presence of jealousy, often without a rational basis.

- Irritability: Individuals who may benefit from Apis exhibit irritability, particularly when unwell.

- Fickleness: There is often a lack of concentration and a tendency to be easily bored or fickle.

Emotional Symptoms: The emotional aspects associated with Apis Mellifica include:

- Sudden Outbursts: Individuals may experience sudden outbursts of tears or anger without apparent provocation.

- Anxiety: There is often anxiety about one's health, particularly regarding minor symptoms.

- Indifference: Apis can be medicated when there is an unusual indifference to loved ones or previously enjoyable activities.

Psychological Symptoms: On a psychological level, Apis Mellifica addresses:

• Inconsistency in Behavior: A tendency towards capriciousness, with rapid changes in mood and behavior.

• Impatience: A marked sense of impatience, finding it hard to wait or remain calm in situations requiring patience.

• Claustrophobia: A fear of closed spaces or feeling trapped can significantly indicate Apis.

Physical Symptoms: The physical indications for Apis Mellifica are diverse and strongly linked to inflammatory responses:

• Skin Conditions: Ap is convenient for conditions like hives, insect bites, and other skin eruptions that are red, swollen, and accompanied by stinging pain, often improving with cold applications.

- Edema: It is a crucial remedy for different types of edema, mainly when the swelling is puffy, tender, and worsens with heat.

- Acute Inflammations: Conditions such as acute sore throat, conjunctivitis, and cystitis, characterized by burning and stinging pain, are within the therapeutic spectrum of Apis.

- Allergic Reactions: Apis is often turned to for acute allergic reactions, especially when there is swelling of the affected area, similar to a bee sting.

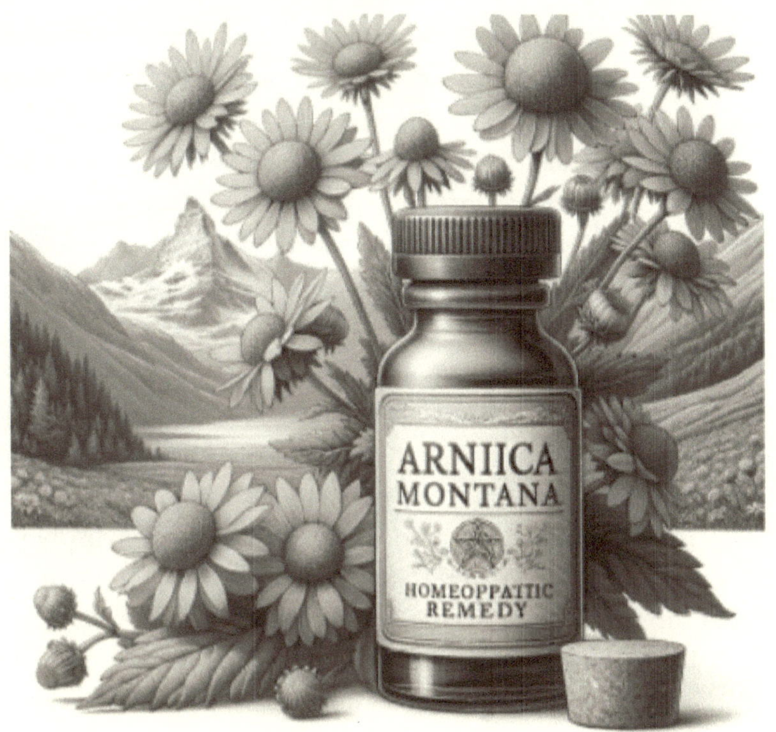

Arnica Montana:

Introduction: Arnica montana is a widely used homeopathic remedy derived from a plant native to Europe and Siberia, with bright yellow, daisy-like flowers. It's primarily sought for its potential in treating physical ailments such as bruising, swelling, and pain resulting from minor injuries.

Homeopathic Preparation and Application: Arnica is prepared through serial dilution and succussion, a cornerstone process in homeopathy believed to increase the remedy's potency. It's available in various forms, including pellets, gels, ointments, and creams, and is commonly used for conditions like postoperative recovery, muscle soreness, arthritic pain, and the aftermath of trauma.

Mental Symptoms: Arnica is often considered in homeopathy for individuals displaying specific mental or cognitive symptoms following trauma or injury:

- Denial of Injury: A tendency to underestimate one's injuries or ailments, often insisting that they are acceptable when not.

- Fear of Contact: An exacerbated fear or anxiety about being touched or approached, likely due to the pain associated with their injury.

- Restlessness: An unease or agitation that makes it difficult for the individual to remain still, even when movement exacerbates their pain.

Emotional Symptoms: The emotional state of a person requiring Arnica can be pretty distinctive, characterized by:

- Irritability and Anguish: There may be marked irritability or distress, especially if attempts are made to offer help or are questioned about their well-being.

- Desire for Solitude: A pronounced wish to be left alone, often rejecting help or asserting that they do not need assistance, even when it's evident they do.

- Mood Swings: Some individuals might experience sudden emotional shifts, ranging from anger to indifference, particularly in the aftermath of trauma.

Psychological Symptoms: Arnica can also address certain psychological aspects that might arise due to physical or emotional trauma:

- Trauma and Shock: The psychological impact of shock or trauma, manifesting as a kind of mental 'bruising,' mirroring the physical symptoms Arnica is known to treat.

- Avoidance Behaviors: An inclination to avoid dealing with the trauma or its implications, which might include avoiding medical treatment or help from others.

- Cognitive Dissonance: Holding conflicting beliefs, such as recognizing the need for recovery while simultaneously denying the severity of one's condition.

Physical Symptoms: Beyond the well-known applications for bruising and swelling, Arnica's physical indications may include a broader spectrum of symptoms:

- Severe Bruising and Swelling: For more significant traumas leading to deep tissue bruising and swelling, where the affected area is incredibly tender and sore.

- Post-Surgical Recovery: Used to potentially reduce the effects of soft tissue damage following surgical procedures.

- Muscle Fatigue: For profound muscle fatigue resulting from overexertion, beyond ordinary soreness.

- Joint Pain: While less common, Arnica may be indicated for joint pain stemming from injury rather than chronic conditions like arthritis.

- Head Injuries: In cases of head injuries or concussions, Arnica is sometimes considered to help manage swelling and bruising of the brain or scalp.

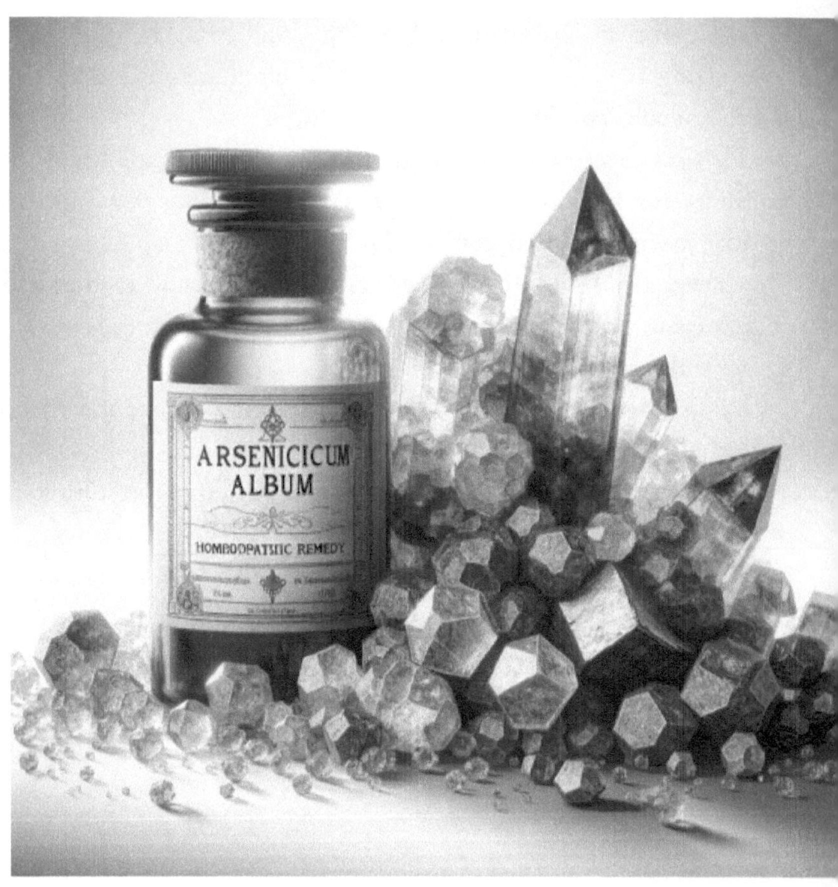
ARSENICICUM
ALBUM

HOMŒOPATHIC REMEDY

Arsenicum Album:

Introduction: Arsenicum Album, commonly known as Arsenic Alb, is a fundamental homeopathic remedy derived from the metallic element arsenic. It's extensively utilized in homeopathy for its potential to address a wide array of health issues, particularly those involving anxiety, restlessness, and digestive disorders. The remedy is reputed for treating symptoms that manifest with burning sensations and are often relieved by warmth.

Homeopathic Preparation and Application: In line with homeopathic principles, Arsenicum Album is prepared through a meticulous process of dilution and succussion. This process imbues the substance with therapeutic properties while eliminating toxic effects. Arsenicum Album is employed in the management of various conditions, including anxiety disorders, gastrointestinal complaints, skin conditions, and respiratory issues.

Mental Symptoms: Arsenicum Album is particularly noted for its action on the cognitive and emotional spheres, characterized by:

- Anxiety and Fear: Individuals who may benefit from Arsenicum Album often experience intense anxiety, especially about health and security, accompanied by fears of death or being left alone.

- Restlessness: A profound sense of restlessness and unease, particularly at night, is a hallmark of the remedy's mental symptomatology.

- Perfectionism: A tendency towards fastidiousness and a need for order and control is standard, often stemming from underlying anxieties.

Emotional Symptoms: The emotional landscape of those requiring Arsenicum Album can be complex, involving:

- Insecurity: Feelings of insecurity and vulnerability, leading to dependency on others for reassurance.

- Despair: Intense feelings of despair, particularly in the face of illness or financial insecurity.

- Irritability: A marked irritability and impatience, especially when feeling unwell or under stress.

Psychological Symptoms: On a psychological level, Arsenicum Album addresses symptoms such as:

- Obsessive Thoughts: Persistent worrying and obsessive thoughts about health, safety, and order.

- Fear of Isolation: A deep-seated fear of being alone or abandoned, often leading to clinginess.

- Control Issues: A need to control one's environment and situations, partly as a coping mechanism for underlying anxieties.

Physical Symptoms: Arsenicum Album's physical indications are diverse, often involving burning pains and symptoms improved by heat:

- Digestive Disorders: It is frequently indicated for gastritis, food poisoning, and digestive disturbances characterized by burning pain, vomiting, and diarrhea.

- Respiratory Issues: Useful in treating colds, coughs, and asthma, especially when accompanied by restlessness and anxiety.

- Skin Conditions: Effective for various skin issues, including eczema, psoriasis, and urticaria, mainly when burning symptoms are improved by heat.

- General Malaise: Symptoms like fever, chills, and general weakness, where the individual feels better with warmth and becomes restless or anxious at night.

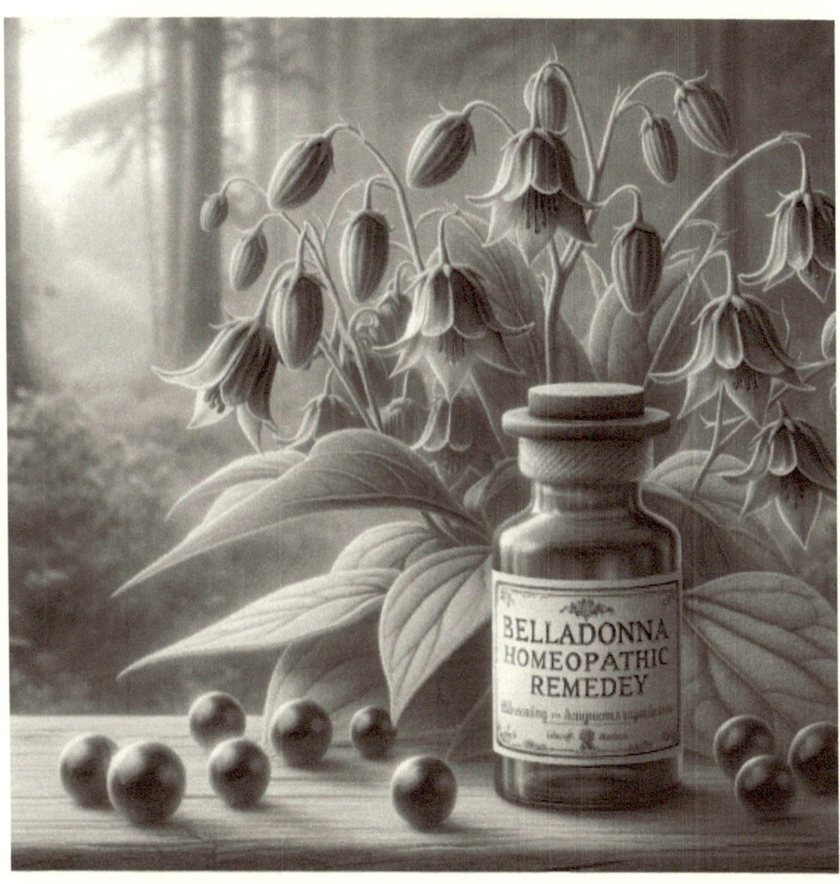

Belladonna:

Introduction: Belladonna, or Deadly Nightshade, is a critical homeopathic remedy derived from a plant native to parts of Europe, North Africa, and Western Asia. Known for its striking bell-shaped flowers and potent berries, Belladonna has a long history in medicine and folklore. In homeopathy, it is renowned for its effectiveness in treating conditions with sudden onset, characterized by fever, inflammation, and throbbing pain.

Homeopathic Preparation and Application: Belladonna is prepared through serial dilution and succussion, ensuring its safety and enhancing its therapeutic potential in line with homeopathic principles. It is commonly indicated for acute conditions such as high fever, earache, sore throat, headaches, and symptoms of heatstroke, where the individual exhibits redness, heat, and pulsating pain.

Mental Symptoms: Belladonna's mental and cognitive symptomatology includes:

- Delirium: Periods of intense excitement or delirium, often accompanied by vivid hallucinations.

- Agitation: A state of heightened agitation or restlessness where the person may lash out or attempt to escape perceived threats.

- Fearfulness: An irrational fear of imaginary things, leading to terror or panic.

Emotional Symptoms: The emotional profile for Belladonna can encompass:

- Mood Swings: Rapid and intense mood swings, from aggressive outbursts to moments of delight or laughter.

- Sensitivity: Heightened sensitivity to external stimuli, such as light, noise, and touch, often exacerbating distress.

- Impulsiveness: Acting on impulses without consideration of consequences, driven by the acute state Belladonna addresses.

Psychological Symptoms: Psychologically, Belladonna may be suited for:

- Confusion: Confusion or disorientation, struggling to differentiate between reality and illusion.

- Suspiciousness: Paranoid or suspicious attitudes towards others, even in familiar settings.

- Hyperalertness: An exaggerated sense of alertness, overreacting to minor stimuli.

Physical Symptoms: Belladonna is particularly effective in treating physical symptoms such as:

- Fever: Sudden, intense fevers with burning heat, red face, and cold extremities, where the person may feel delirious or semi-conscious.

- Inflammatory Conditions: Acute inflammatory reactions, such as red, hot, swollen skin or throbbing pain in affected areas.

- Headaches and Migraines: Severe, pulsating headaches and migraines, often exacerbated by light, noise, or jarring movements.

- Earaches and Sore Throats: Intense, sharp earaches and sore throats with constriction and swallowing difficulties.

- Eye Conditions: Inflammatory eye conditions with redness, dryness, and burning sensation.

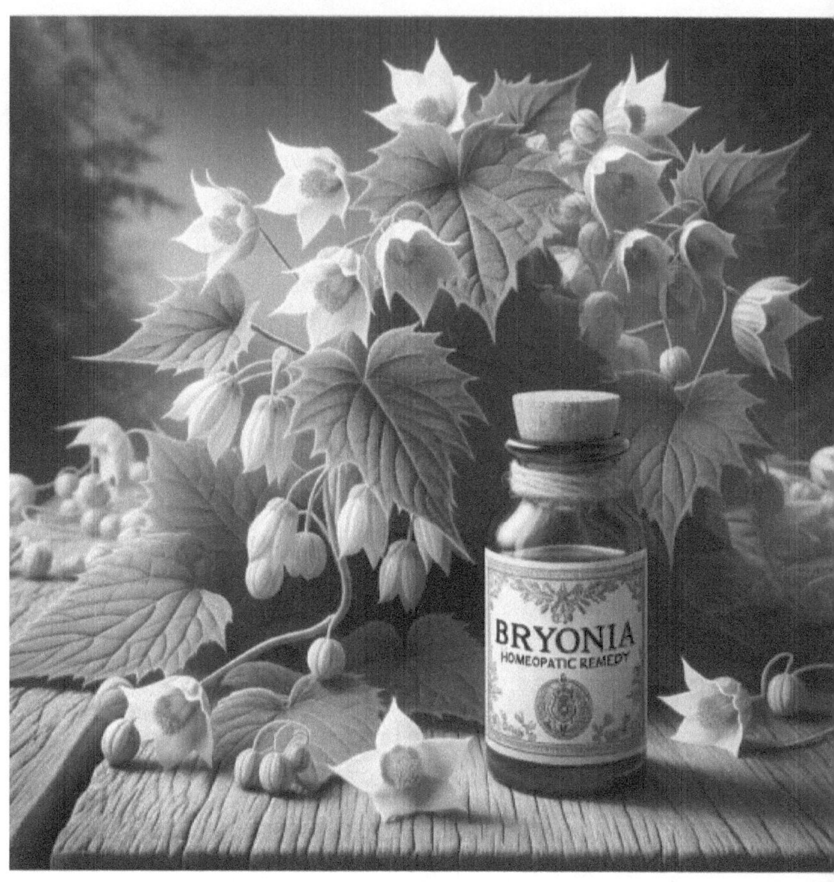

Bryonia:

Introduction: Bryonia, derived from the root of the Bryonia alba plant, also known as white bryony or wild hops, is a highly esteemed homeopathic remedy. It is notably recognized for its efficacy in treating inflammation, dryness, and a strong desire for stability and minimal movement. Bryonia is often the remedy for acute conditions such as dry coughs, joint pain, and gastrointestinal issues, where symptoms worsen with the slightest motion.

Homeopathic Preparation and Application: Through the traditional homeopathic process of dilution and succussion, Bryonia is prepared in a manner that enhances its healing qualities while ensuring safety for therapeutic use. This remedy is most commonly indicated for conditions with dryness, such as dry mucous membranes, and for situations where any movement exacerbates the symptoms, requiring the patient to remain still for relief.

Mental Symptoms: Bryonia addresses several mental and cognitive symptoms, including:

- Irritability: A notable irritability and desire to be left alone, especially when disturbed.

- Anxiety about the Future: Worry or anxiety about the future, often related to financial or health concerns.

- Desire for Stability: A strong preference for remaining stationary, with an aversion to change due to the discomfort it causes.

Emotional Symptoms: The emotional characteristics associated with Bryonia encompass:

- Anger from Disturbance: A tendency to become angry or upset when required to move or when disturbed.

- Moodiness: Sudden mood changes, particularly towards negativity when in pain or discomfort.

- Fear of Motion: An emotional resistance or fear of moving due to exacerbating symptoms.

Psychological Symptoms: Psychologically, Bryonia is suited for:

- Overwhelming from Physical Symptoms: Feelings of being overwhelmed by physical symptoms, leading to a desire for stillness.

- Stress from Immobility: Psychological stress is associated with the inability to move freely without pain.

- Fixation on Symptoms: A preoccupation with one's physical symptoms, leading to persistent worry and negativity.

Physical Symptoms: Bryonia is particularly effective in treating a range of physical symptoms:

- Joint Pain: Stiff, painful joints that feel worse with the slightest movement and better with rest.

- Dry Coughs: Painful, dry coughs that worsen with movement and deep breathing, often requiring the person to hold their chest for relief.

- Headaches: Bursting, throbbing headaches that worsen with movement and improve with pressure or lying on the painful side.

- Constipation: Dry, hard stools and constipation with no desire to drink water despite dryness.

- Fever: Fevers where the patient feels hot, dry, and irritable, wanting to remain perfectly still to avoid aggravating symptoms.

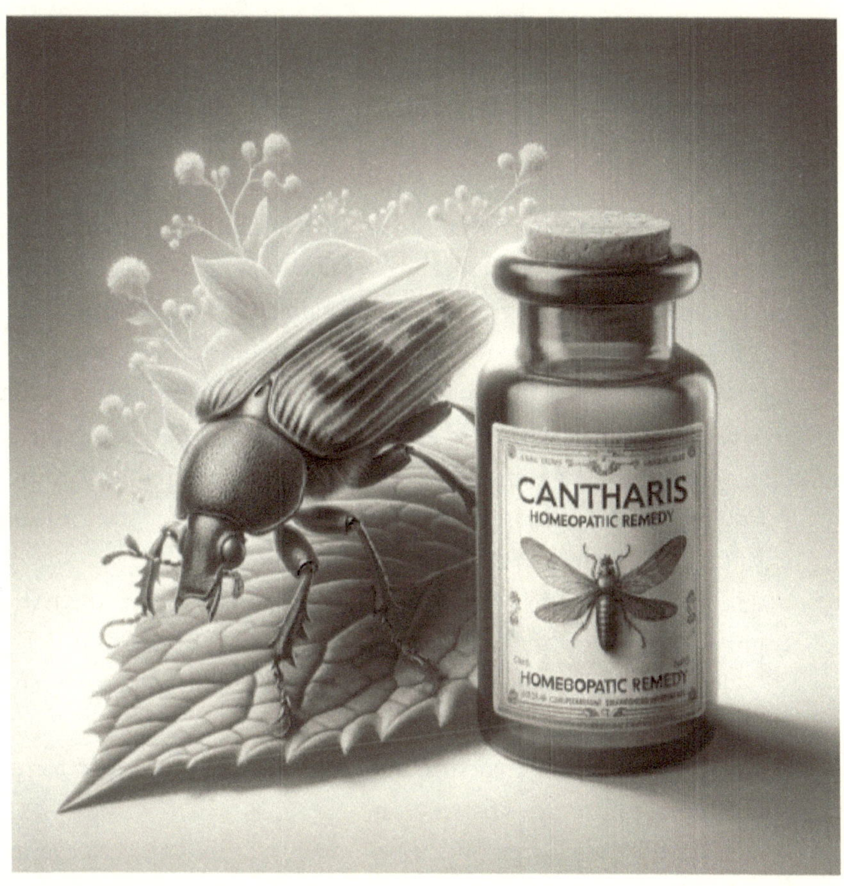
CANTHARIS
HOMEOPATIC REMEDY
HOMEOPATIC REMEDY

Cantharis:

Introduction: Cantharis, known as the Spanish Fly, is derived from the Lytta vesicatoria beetle. This homeopathic remedy is renowned for treating intense burning sensations and inflammation, particularly of the urinary tract and skin. Cantharis is often the remedy for acute cystitis, burns, and scalds, relieving the stinging pain and promoting healing.

Homeopathic Preparation and Application: Through the homeopathic process of dilution and succussion, Cantharis is prepared in a way that maximizes its healing potential while mitigating the toxic effects found in its natural state. It is primarily indicated for conditions involving burning pain, such as severe sunburns, urinary tract infections with painful urination, and blistering skin eruptions.

Mental Symptoms: Cantharis may address specific mental and cognitive symptoms, including:

- Restlessness: An acute sense of restlessness and agitation, often due to the intensity of physical symptoms.

- Irritability: Heightened irritability and a low tolerance for pain, contributing to a sense of frustration.

- Anxiety: Anxiety about health, mainly related to the severity of burning sensations and the potential for worsening conditions.

Emotional Symptoms: The emotional profile for Cantharis includes:

- Impatience: A marked impatience stemming from the discomfort and pain of symptoms.

- Desperation: Feelings of desperation or despair due to intense pain or the distressing nature of symptoms.

- Emotional Sensitivity: Increased emotional sensitivity, where physical discomfort significantly affects mood and emotional well-being.

Psychological Symptoms: Psychologically, Cantharis can be suited for:

- Fear of Water: Due to painful urination, there may be a fear or aversion to drinking water or other liquids.

- Obsession with Symptoms: A preoccupation with one's symptoms, notably the burning sensations, leading to constant concern and monitoring.

- Concentration Difficulties: Challenges with focusing or maintaining attention due to the distraction of severe discomfort.

Physical Symptoms: Cantharis is particularly effective in treating a range of physical symptoms:

- Urinary Tract Infections: Intense burning and cutting pain before, during, and after urination, often with a frequent urge to urinate.

- Burns and Scalds: Second-degree burns with blistering, where the skin exhibits raw, burning pain that seems to be relieved by cold applications.

- Skin Eruptions: Blistering skin eruptions that mimic the effects of burns, with intense burning and itching.

- Sunburn: Severe sunburn with blistering and stinging pain, where the skin is hot to the touch and extremely sensitive.

- Gastritis: Inflammation of the stomach lining presenting with burning pain, possibly exacerbated by consuming certain foods or beverages.

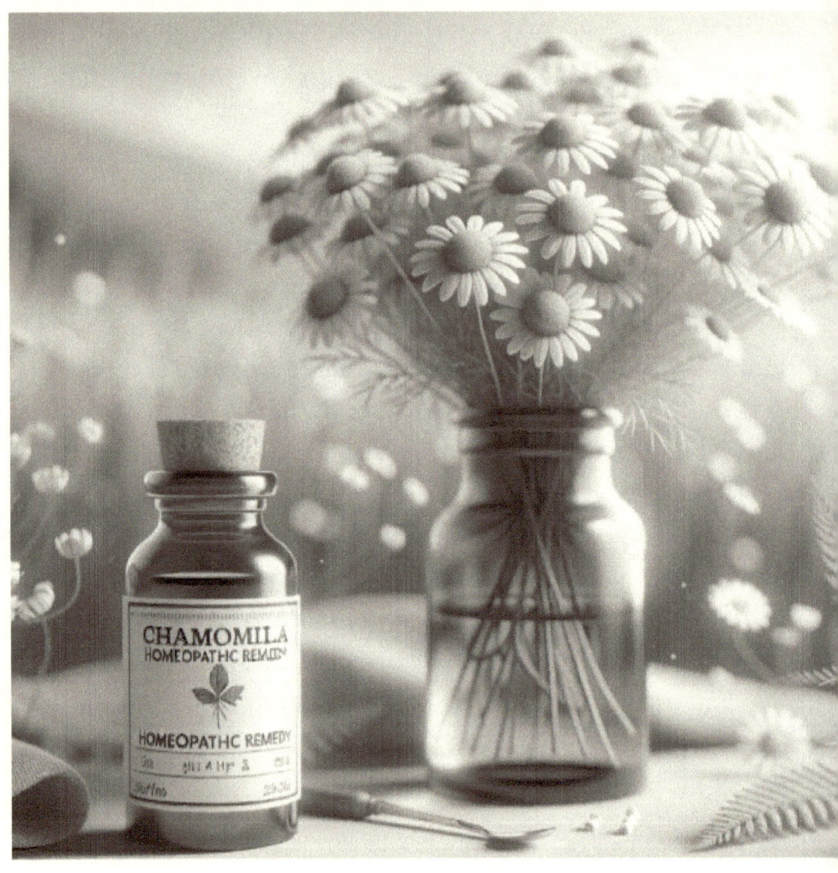
CHAMOMILA
HOMEOPATHIC REMEDY
HOMEOPATHIC REMEDY

Chamomilla:

Introduction: Chamomilla, derived from the Chamomile plant, is a well-regarded homeopathic remedy known for its calming and soothing properties. It is particularly valued in homeopathy for addressing symptoms associated with irritability, infant teething, and sleep disturbances. Chamomilla is often the go-to remedy for patients who exhibit extreme sensitivity to pain and an irritable temperament.

Homeopathic Preparation and Application: Through the homeopathic methodology of dilution and succussion, Chamomilla is prepared in a manner that enhances its therapeutic benefits while ensuring safety. This remedy is most commonly used for acute conditions with sudden onset of intense symptoms, such as colicky pain, teething discomfort in children, and extreme irritability and restlessness.

Mental Symptoms: Chamomilla can help alleviate a range of mental and cognitive symptoms, including:

- Hypersensitivity: An increased sensitivity to all impressions, leading to overreactions to stimuli.

- Impatience: A pronounced sense of impatience, with a tendency to demand immediate attention or relief.

- Frustration: High frustration levels, especially when comfort or relief is not quickly forthcoming.

Emotional Symptoms: The emotional characteristics associated with Chamomilla include:

- Irritability: Extreme irritability, where the individual may be inconsolable or prone to anger over minor issues.

- Mood Swings: Sudden and intense mood swings, often from a calm state to one of agitation or vice versa.

- Tearfulness: An inclination towards being tearful or crying, especially in response to pain or discomfort.

Psychological Symptoms: On a psychological level, Chamomilla is indicated for:

- Oversensitivity to Pain: An exaggerated response to pain, where the perceived intensity is much greater than the actual stimulus.

- Restlessness: Psychological restlessness that manifests as an inability to stay calm or focused, often due to discomfort or pain.

- Demanding Behavior: The person may exhibit demanding or hard-to-please behavior, often as a coping mechanism for the underlying discomfort.

Physical Symptoms: Chamomilla is particularly effective in addressing physical symptoms such as:

- Teething Pain: Relief for infants and young children experiencing intense pain and irritability during teething, often accompanied by drooling and swollen gums.

- Colic and Digestive Discomfort: Useful in treating colicky pain, characterized by intense abdominal discomfort, gas, and bloating, especially in infants.

- Sleep Disturbances: Helps alleviate sleeplessness and restlessness at night, particularly when associated with pain or discomfort.

- Earache: Effective for acute ear pain, especially when it's intense and the person exhibits extreme irritability.

- Menstrual Cramps: Can relieve severe menstrual cramps that cause irritability and restlessness.

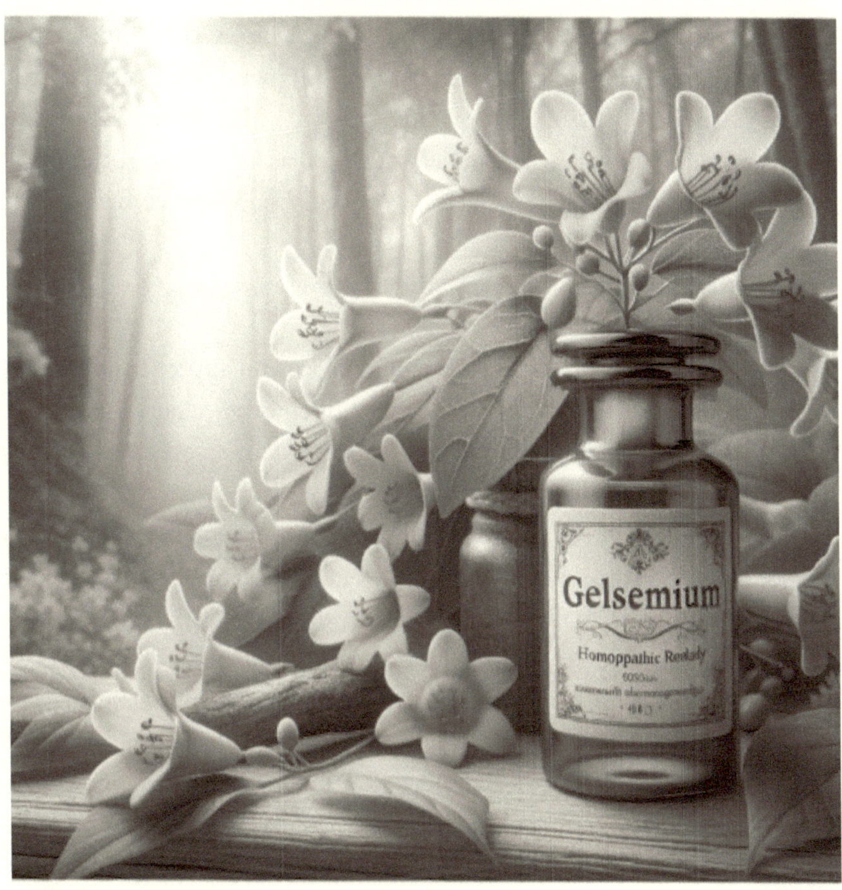

Gelsemium:

Introduction: Gelsemium, derived from the yellow jasmine plant Gelsemium sempervirens, is a prominent homeopathic remedy for treating nervous disorders, anxiety, and flu-like symptoms. It is beneficial for conditions that arise from anticipation, fear, or shock, leading to physical and mental paralysis. Gelsemium is the remedy of choice for individuals who experience weakness, dizziness, and trembling from emotional or physical stress.

Homeopathic Preparation and Application: Gelsemium is prepared through the homeopathic process of dilution and succussion, enhancing its healing properties while ensuring safety. This remedy is commonly recommended for acute anxiety states, fear of public speaking, stage fright, and the onset of flu or fever where the patient feels heavy, sluggish, and dull.

Mental Symptoms: Gelsemium addresses a variety of mental and cognitive symptoms, such as:

- Anticipation Anxiety: Intense anxiety and apprehension before an upcoming event, such as an exam or public performance.

- Mental Fatigue: A sense of dullness and sluggishness in mental processes, with difficulty concentrating.

- Fear of Loss of Control: Fear that they might lose control or that something terrible will happen, leading to avoidance behaviors.

Emotional Symptoms: The emotional aspects linked with Gelsemium include:

- Timidity: A timid nature, lacking confidence in social situations or when facing new challenges.

- Emotional Withdrawal: A tendency to withdraw or shut down emotionally in response to stress or anxiety.

- Sense of Apprehension: A pervasive dread or apprehension about the future or unknown outcomes.

Psychological Symptoms: Psychologically, Gelsemium is suited for:

- Overwhelming Feelings of being overwhelmed by responsibilities or upcoming events, leading to a desire to escape or hide.

- Indecision: Difficulty making decisions due to a lack of confidence and overwhelming anxiety.

- Despondency: A state of hopelessness or depression triggered by fear or anticipation of stressful events.

Physical Symptoms: Gelsemium effectively treats physical symptoms such as:

- Flu-like Symptoms: General malaise, weakness, and trembling with fever, often without thirst.

- Headaches: Dull, severe headaches, especially at the base of the skull, extending to the neck and shoulders.

- Muscle Weakness: Profound muscular weakness and fatigue, making even small tasks seem daunting.

- Dizziness and Vertigo: Sensations of dizziness and vertigo, often related to emotional stress or anxiety.

- Vision Problems: Blurred vision or difficulty focusing, associated with nervous tension or fatigue.

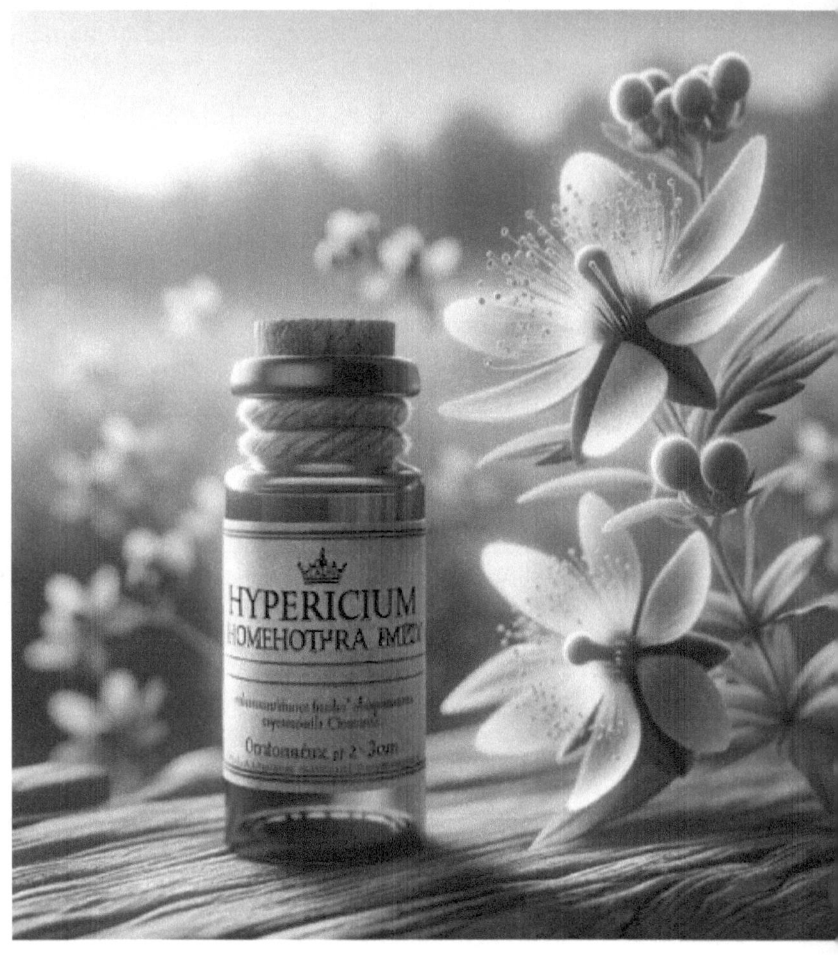

Hypericum:

Introduction: Hypericum, commonly known as St. John's Wort, is a well-regarded homeopathic remedy with a rich history in herbal medicine. In homeopathy, Hypericum is primarily used for its exceptional ability to treat nerve injuries, especially in areas rich in nerve endings. It is the remedy of choice for conditions such as crushed fingers, spinal injuries, and the effects of shock and trauma on the nervous system.

Homeopathic Preparation and Application: Through the homeopathic process of dilution and succussion, Hypericum is prepared in a way that maximizes its healing potential while ensuring safety. This remedy is particularly effective for injuries to nerve-rich areas, post-surgical pain, dental procedures, and the prevention and treatment of tetanus.

Mental Symptoms: Hypericum can help alleviate mental and cognitive symptoms associated with nerve injuries, including:

- Anxiety Following Injury: Anxiety or nervousness following an injury, mainly when there is nerve damage involved.

- Effects of Shock: Mental and emotional effects of shock from injuries, with symptoms such as confusion or disorientation.

- Mood Changes: Mood changes post-injury, especially irritability or frustration due to pain or restricted mobility.

Emotional Symptoms: The emotional profile for Hypericum includes:

- Despondency: Despondency or despair following severe injuries, especially when recovery is slow.

- Heightened Sensitivity: Increased emotional sensitivity post-injury, where the individual may react strongly to what they perceive as a lack of empathy.

- Fear of Nerve Pain: Fear or anxiety about enduring nerve pain or the possibility of chronic pain conditions developing.

Psychological Symptoms: Psychologically, Hypericum is indicated for:

- Trauma Impact: The psychological impact of physical trauma, including flashbacks or recurrent memories of the injury event.

- Concentration Difficulties: Difficulty concentrating or maintaining focus due to persistent pain or discomfort from nerve damage.

- Stress from Immobility: Psychological stress associated with immobility or reduced physical function due to nerve injuries.

Physical Symptoms: Hypericum is particularly effective in treating physical symptoms such as:

- Nerve Pain: Sharp, shooting pains along nerve pathways or numbness and tingling in affected areas.

- Injuries to Extremities: Injuries to fingers, toes, and spinal injuries where there is significant nerve involvement.

- Post-Surgical Nerve Pain: Pain following surgical procedures, particularly in areas with dense nerve distribution.

- Dental Pain: Pain from dental procedures or tooth extractions, especially when the pain radiates along nerve pathways.

- Puncture Wounds: Treatment of puncture wounds where there is a risk of nerve damage or tetanus.

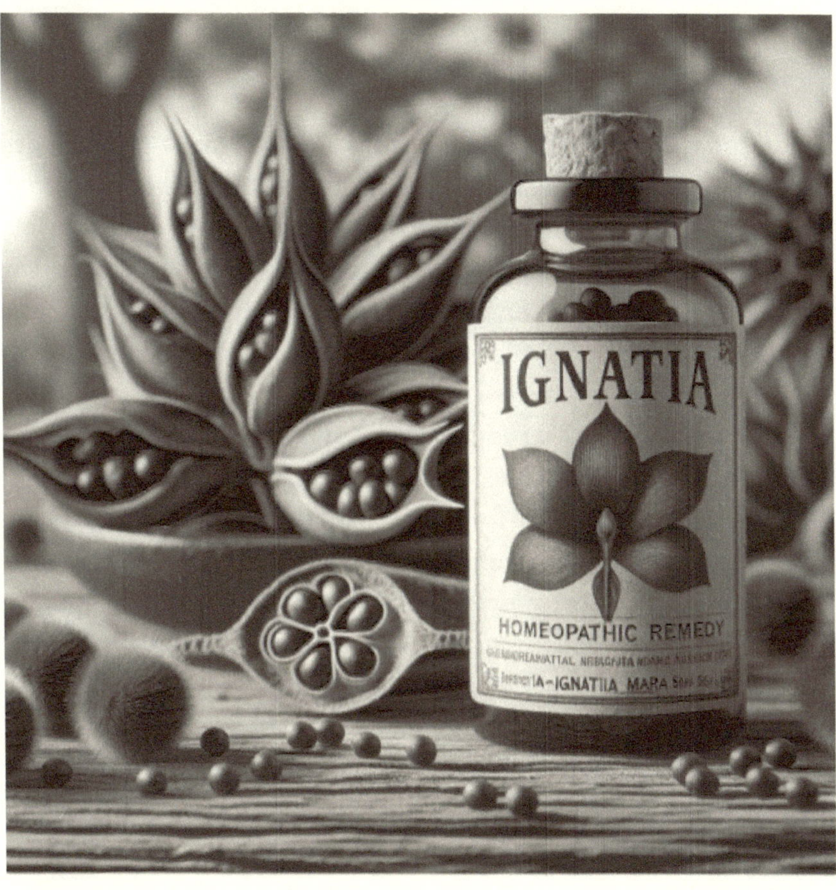
IGNATIA
HOMEOPATHIC REMEDY

Ignatia:

Introduction: Ignatia, more formally known as Ignatia Amara, is derived from the seeds of the St. Ignatius bean tree, native to the Philippines and other parts of Southeast Asia. This homeopathic remedy is highly valued for its ability to address emotional and psychological issues, particularly those related to grief, loss, and acute emotional shock. It is often called the "homeopathic Prozac" for its effectiveness in dealing with various forms of emotional distress.

Homeopathic Preparation and Application: Prepared through the process of dilution and succussion, Ignatia is rendered safe and therapeutically potent for homeopathic use. It is most commonly recommended for individuals experiencing acute emotional reactions, such as intense grief, anxiety, or the aftermath of a shock. Symptoms that respond well to Ignatia often have a paradoxical quality, such as a sore throat that feels better when swallowing or a mood that shifts rapidly from laughter to tears.

Mental Symptoms: The mental and cognitive symptoms addressed by Ignatia include:

- Contradictory Behavior: A notable feature is the presence of contradictory behaviors or feelings, often changing rapidly.

- Concentration Issues: Difficulty focusing or concentrating, often due to emotional turmoil.

- Sensitivity: An increased sensitivity to emotional and physical stimuli, with a tendency to startle easily.

Emotional Symptoms: Ignatia's influence on the emotional state is marked by:

- Mood Variability: Swift mood changes from intense sadness to moments of relief, often without apparent cause.

- Suppressed Grief: Deep grief or sorrow that may be internalized, leading to physical symptoms.

- Sighing: Frequent sighing as a physical manifestation of emotional stress or sadness.

Psychological Symptoms: Psychologically, Ignatia can be beneficial for:

- Acute Emotional Shock: The aftermath of a sudden emotional shock, such as the loss of a loved one or the end of a close relationship.

- Internal Conflict: Struggles with internal conflicts, often related to suppressed emotions or unexpressed feelings.

- Sensation of a Lump in the Throat: The feeling of a lump in the throat that cannot be swallowed, often associated with unsaid or swallowed emotions.

Physical Symptoms: Ignatia is adept at addressing physical symptoms associated with emotional states, such as:

- Headaches: Tension headaches or migraines triggered by emotional stress or conflict.

- Sleep Disturbances: Difficulty falling asleep or frequent waking, often due to an overactive mind or emotional distress.

- Muscular Twitches: Involuntary muscular cramps or spasms, particularly in the face or limbs, related to nervous tension.

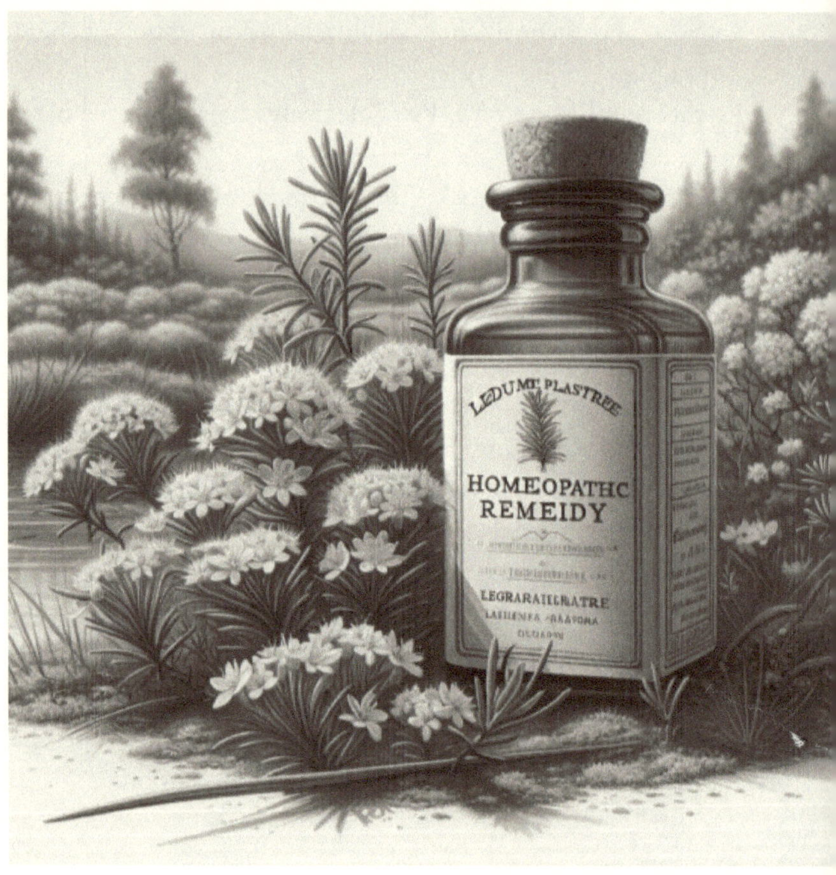

Ledum:

Introduction: Ledum, known fully as Ledum Palustre and commonly referred to as Wild Rosemary, is a homeopathic remedy derived from a perennial, evergreen shrub found in the cooler regions of the Northern Hemisphere. In homeopathy, Ledum is esteemed for its efficacy in treating puncture wounds, insect bites, and various conditions associated with coldness, swelling, and bruising.

Homeopathic Preparation and Application: Through the meticulous process of dilution and succussion, Ledum is prepared for homeopathic use, ensuring its safety and enhancing its healing properties. It is predominantly used for injuries that feel cold to the touch and are relieved by cold applications, such as ice packs. Conditions commonly treated with Ledum include puncture wounds from nails or needles, animal and insect bites, and the early stages of gout.

Mental Symptoms: While Ledum is primarily known for its physical applications, it can also address specific mental and cognitive symptoms:

- Irritability: A tendency towards irritability and frustration, especially when in pain.

- Restlessness: An underlying sense of restlessness that may accompany physical discomfort.

- Lack of Concentration: Difficulty focusing or concentrating, possibly due to discomfort or pain from injuries.

Emotional Symptoms: The emotional aspects related to the use of Ledum include:

- Anxiety: Anxiety related to health concerns, particularly after receiving a puncture wound or insect bite.

- Mood Swings: Sudden mood changes, potentially triggered by physical symptoms or the stress of injury.

- Sensitivity: Emotional sensitivity, particularly in response to physical ailments.

Psychological Symptoms: Ledum may be beneficial for addressing psychological responses such as:

- Fear of Disease: Fear or worry about potential diseases resulting from wounds or bites.

- Disproportionate Reactions: Overly strong emotional reactions to minor physical injuries.

- Obsession with Injuries: Preoccupation with the injury and its possible complications.

Physical Symptoms: Ledum is particularly effective for a range of physical symptoms:

- Puncture Wounds: Ideal for treating puncture wounds that exhibit coldness and are relieved by cold applications.

- Insect Bites: Effective for mosquito, spider, and other insect bites that swell, turn purple, and feel cold.

- Joint Pain: Used in treating gout and rheumatism, especially when the affected area is cold and feels better with cold applications.

- Bruising and Swelling: Useful for bruises that are cold to the touch and for swelling from sprains or other injuries.

- Eye Injuries: Ledum can be indicated for black eyes and other eye injuries, particularly when the affected area feels better with cold compresses.

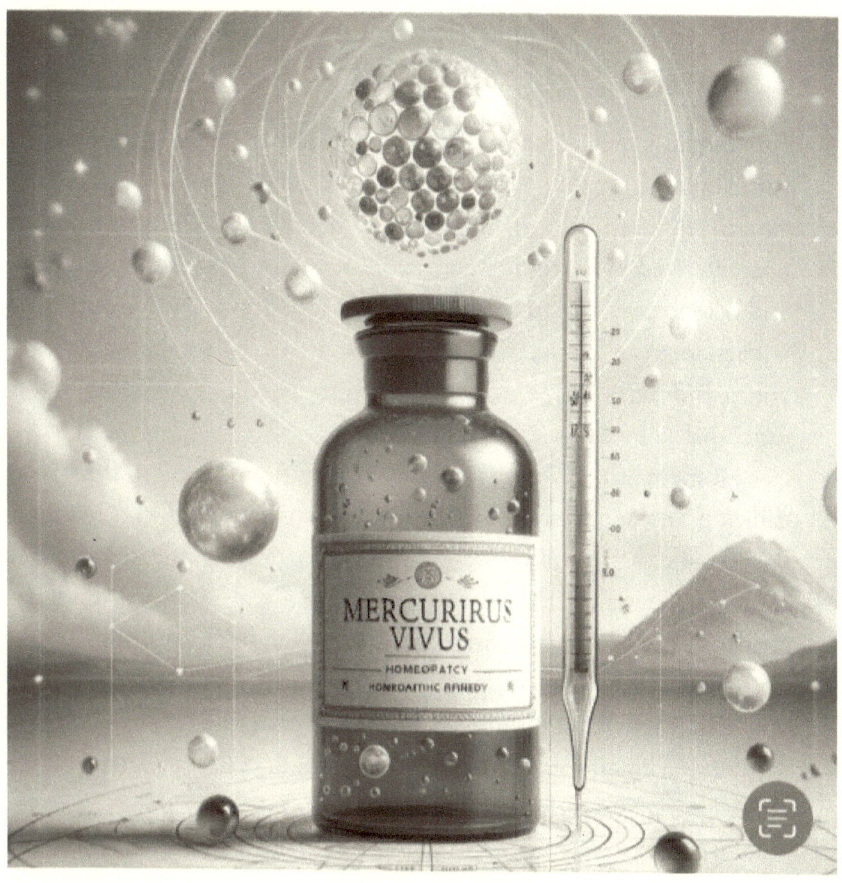
MERCURIRUS
VIVUS
HOMEOPATCY
HOMEOPATHIC REMEDY

Mercurius Vivus:

Introduction: Mercurius Vivus, commonly called Mercury, is a fundamental homeopathic remedy derived from mercury. It is extensively used in homeopathy to address a wide range of conditions characterized by extreme fluctuations in symptoms, excessive salivation, and a tendency towards infection and inflammation. Mercurius Vivus is particularly effective for treating issues related to the mouth, throat, and glandular systems, where symptoms are often worse at night and exacerbated by temperature changes.

Homeopathic Preparation and Application: Through the process of dilution and succussion, Mercurius Vivus is prepared in a manner that ensures its therapeutic efficacy while neutralizing the toxic effects of elemental mercury. This remedy is commonly prescribed for conditions such as sore throats, dental problems, glandular swellings, and skin eruptions, where there is significant night-time aggravation and a general worsening of symptoms due to warmth or dampness.

Mental Symptoms: Mercurius Vivus addresses a variety of mental and cognitive symptoms, including:

- Restlessness: A marked sense of restlessness and unease, particularly at night.

- Anxiety: Anxiety about one's health, often accompanied by a lack of confidence in recovery.

- Suspiciousness: A tendency towards distrustfulness or suspiciousness, even in familiar environments.

Emotional Symptoms: The emotional profile for Mercurius Vivus includes:

- Mood Swings: Rapid and unpredictable changes in mood, often without a clear trigger.

- Irritability: Heightened irritability, especially in response to physical discomfort or worsening symptoms.

- Despondency: Feelings of hopelessness or despair, particularly during the peak of symptoms.

Psychological Symptoms: Psychologically, Mercurius Vivus is suited for:

- Fear of Losing Control: An underlying fear of losing control over one's health or circumstances.

- Indecisiveness: Difficult decision-making, often due to a lack of clarity or fluctuating opinions.

- Memory Challenges: Struggles with memory and concentration, exacerbated by the physical symptoms.

Physical Symptoms: Mercurius Vivus is especially effective in treating physical symptoms such as:

- Sore Throats: Intense sore throats with excessive salivation, swelling, and redness, worsening at night.

- Dental Issues: Toothaches and gum problems with increased salivation and foul breath.

- Glandular Swelling: Swollen glands, particularly in the neck, with tenderness and sensitivity.

- Skin Eruptions: Weeping skin eruptions sensitive to temperature changes and prone to infection.

- Night Sweats: Profuse sweating at night, which does not bring relief to symptoms.

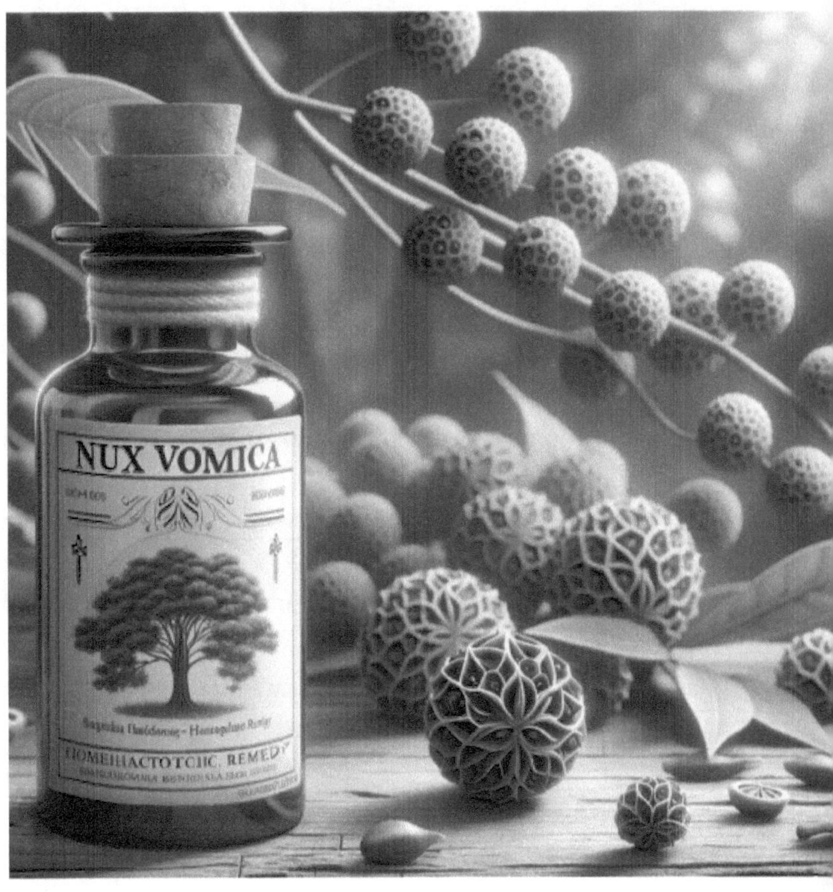

Nux Vomica:

Introduction: Nux Vomica, derived from the seeds of the Strychnine tree native to India and Southeast Asia, is a cornerstone homeopathic remedy known for its effectiveness in treating digestive disturbances, sleeplessness, and conditions stemming from overindulgence or stress. It is particularly suited for individuals who lead a fast-paced, competitive lifestyle, often resorting to stimulants or sedatives to manage their energy levels.

Homeopathic Preparation and Application: Through the process of dilution and succussion, Nux Vomica is prepared in a manner that ensures its therapeutic efficacy while neutralizing the toxic effects of its natural state. This remedy is commonly prescribed for symptoms such as constipation, heartburn, and irritability, significantly when these are exacerbated by stress, lack of sleep, or dietary indiscretions.

Mental Symptoms: Nux Vomica addresses a variety of mental and cognitive symptoms, including:

- Irritability and impatience, especially under stress.

- Competitive and ambitious nature, often leading to overexertion.

- Sensitivity to noise and odors, reflecting a general state of nervous stimulation.

Emotional Symptoms: The emotional profile for Nux Vomica includes:

- Quick to anger, with difficulty tolerating interruption or contradiction.

- Stress and frustration, mainly related to work or personal achievements.

- A tendency toward mood swings influenced by stress or digestive issues.

Psychological Symptoms: Psychologically, Nux Vomica is suited for:

- Stress-related issues, particularly where ambition leads to overwork and burnout.

- Anxiety about health and well-being, often focusing on digestive discomfort or sleep problems.

- A strong desire for stimulants like caffeine or alcohol to maintain energy levels or relieve stress.

Physical Symptoms: Nux Vomica is particularly effective in treating physical symptoms such as:

- Digestive issues, including constipation, heartburn, and bloating, are often related to stress or dietary excess.

- Sleep disturbances, characterized by difficulty falling asleep or waking in the early hours, with the inability to fall back asleep.

- Headaches and migraines, mainly stemming from digestive issues or stress.

- Muscular tension and back pain are often related to stress or long hours spent sitting, especially at a desk or in front of a computer.

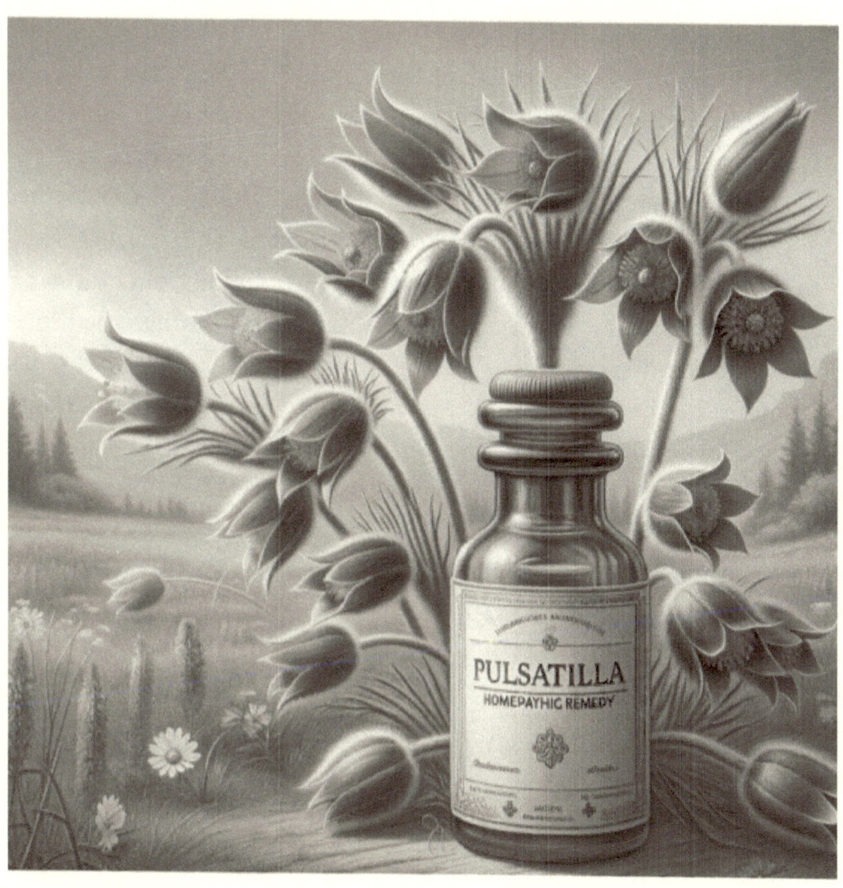

PULSATILLA
HOMEPAYHIC REMEDY

Pulsatilla:

Introduction: Pulsatilla, derived from the Pasque flower (Pulsatilla pratensis), is a critical homeopathic remedy known for its gentle action, particularly effective in treating conditions characterized by changeability, mildness, and emotional vulnerability. It is well-suited for gentle, yielding individuals who crave comfort and reassurance, often showing improvement from fresh air and worsening from heat.

Homeopathic Preparation and Application: Through the process of dilution and succussion, Pulsatilla is prepared in a way that enhances its healing properties while ensuring safety. This remedy is commonly used for conditions such as weepy colds, variegated menstrual disorders, and mood swings, where symptoms are changeable, and the emotional component is pronounced.

Mental Symptoms: Pulsatilla addresses a variety of mental and cognitive symptoms, including:

- Emotional and weepy disposition, especially when seeking attention or comfort.

- Timidity and shyness, with a tendency to feel better in the company of loved ones.

- Changeable moods and indecisiveness, often influenced by emotional states.

Emotional Symptoms: The emotional profile for Pulsatilla includes:

- A need for reassurance and sympathy, often feeling abandoned or alone.

- Jealousy and possessiveness, particularly in close relationships.

- Tendency to cry easily, especially when feeling neglected or misunderstood.

Psychological Symptoms: Psychologically, Pulsatilla is suited for:

- Issues related to dependency and attachment, seeking constant support and validation.

- Fear of abandonment, leading to clingy and possessive behavior.

- Adaptability and impressionability, often influenced by the moods and opinions of others.

Physical Symptoms: Pulsatilla is particularly effective in treating physical symptoms such as:

- Colds and congestion with thick, yellow discharge, improving in open air.

- Menstrual disorders with irregular or delayed cycles, accompanied by mood swings and tearfulness.

- Digestive issues, particularly from rich or fatty foods, with a need for gentle remedies and a preference for cool, fresh air.

- Varicose veins and circulatory problems, often feeling better with gentle movement and excellent applications.

- Styes and eye infections with a thick, yellowish discharge, where symptoms improve with exposure to fresh air.

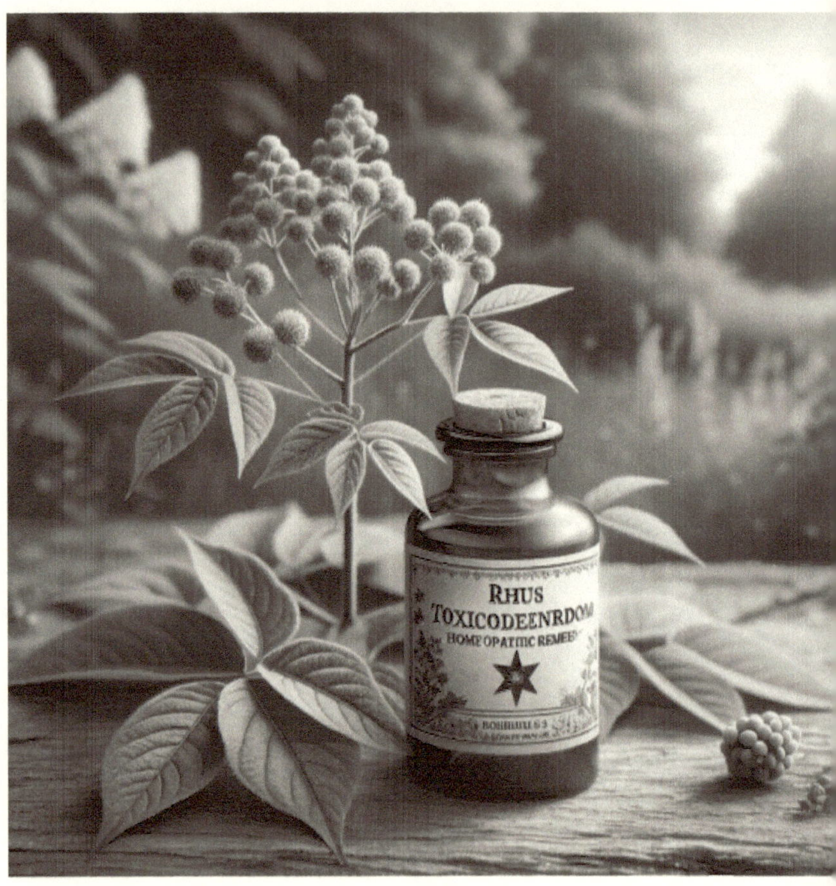

Rhus Toxicodendron:

Introduction: Rhus Toxicodendron, commonly known as Rhus Tox, is a widely used homeopathic remedy derived from the poison ivy plant. It is prominent in homeopathy for its effectiveness in treating stiffness, inflammation, and skin rashes. Rhus Tox is particularly indicated for individuals experiencing musculoskeletal complaints that improve with movement, as well as for various skin conditions resembling poison ivy rashes.

Homeopathic Preparation and Application: In keeping with homeopathic principles, Rhus Tox is meticulously prepared through serial dilution and succussion. This method is believed to enhance the remedy's healing properties while eliminating the toxic effects of the crude substance. It is commonly employed to alleviate symptoms of arthritis, back pain, sprains, strains, and skin conditions with intense itching and blistering.

Mental Symptoms: Rhus Tox may be beneficial for individuals displaying specific mental and cognitive symptoms such as:

• Restlessness and agitation, mainly when physical discomfort is present.

• health anxiety, especially when experiencing chronic pain or skin ailments.

• Irritability stemming from pain or immobility, often leading to frustration over limitations.

Emotional Symptoms: The emotional landscape of those who may benefit from Rhus Tox includes:

• Impatience with the healing process, especially in slow recovery from joint or muscle injuries.

• Discouragement or low spirits when physical conditions impede daily activities.

• A tendency to feel better with distraction and movement despite initial discomfort.

Psychological Symptoms: Rhus Tox addresses several psychological aspects:

• A desire for constant change or movement as a coping mechanism for discomfort.

• Fear of deterioration of physical condition, leading to obsessive concern over health.

• Sensation of being trapped or confined by physical ailments, craving the freedom of movement.

Physical Symptoms: Rhus Tox is highly effective for a range of physical symptoms:

• Joint and Muscle Pain: Excellent for pain and stiffness in joints and muscles, significantly when symptoms improve with gentle movement.

• Skin Afflictions: Useful for treating skin rashes that mimic poison ivy exposure, with intense itching, redness, and blistering.

• Sprains and Strains: Ideal for treating ligament and tendon injuries where initial movement causes pain, but continued movement brings relief.

• Back Pain: Effective for lower back pain that improves with motion, often used for conditions like sciatica or lumbago.

• Flu and Cold Symptoms: Beneficial for flu-like symptoms that involve aching, stiffness, and restlessness, particularly when symptoms are aggravated by cold, damp weather.

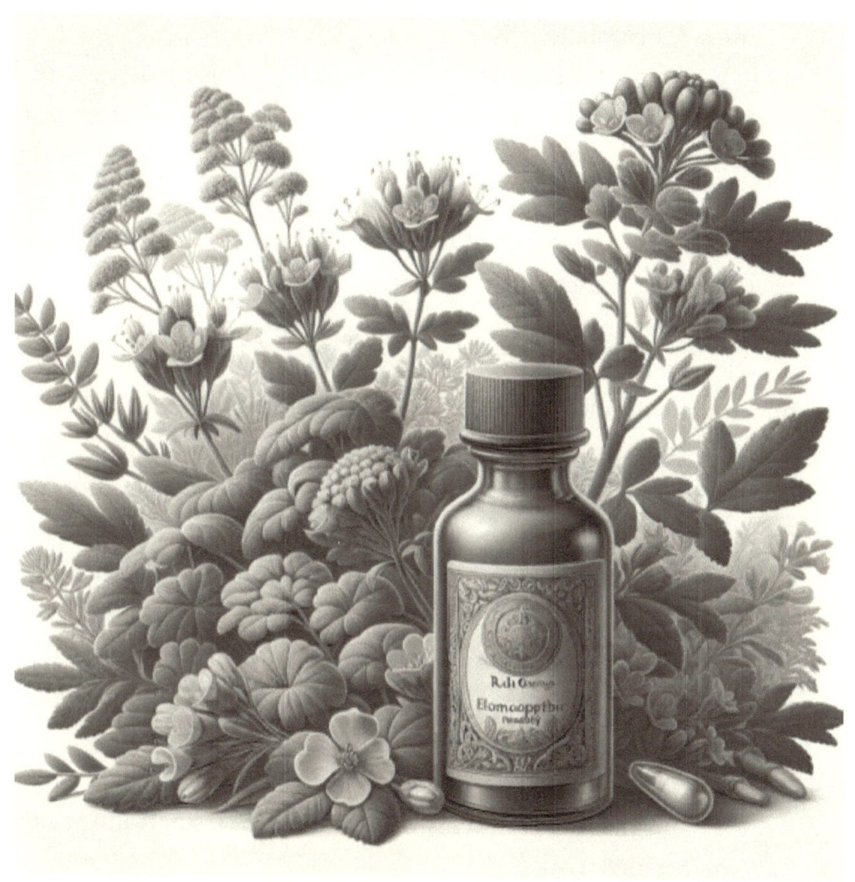

Ruta Graveolens:

Introduction: Ruta Graveolens, commonly known as Ruta or Rue, is a valued homeopathic remedy derived from a perennial herb in the Rutaceae family, native to the Balkan Peninsula but found in various parts of the world. Traditionally used in both herbal and homeopathic medicine, Ruta is renowned for its effectiveness in treating conditions related to the musculoskeletal system, particularly issues involving the tendons, ligaments, and periosteum.

Homeopathic Preparation and Application: In accordance with homeopathic principles, Ruta is meticulously prepared through dilution and succussion. This method enhances the plant's medicinal properties and eliminates toxic side effects. Ruta is primarily employed in treating injuries and strains to the connective tissues, eye strain, and joint problems, particularly when the affected areas feel bruised or achy, and symptoms improve with movement.

Mental Symptoms: While Ruta is predominantly recognized for its physical applications, it can also be beneficial for specific mental and cognitive symptoms associated with overexertion or strain:

- Irritability due to physical discomfort or limitations in movement.
- Mental fatigue, primarily related to eye strain from prolonged focus on detailed work.
- A feeling of dissatisfaction or restlessness when physical ailments prevent routine activities.

Emotional Symptoms: The emotional state of individuals who may benefit from Ruta can include:

- Frustration and impatience with the healing process, especially in slow recovery from tendon or ligament injuries.
- Despondency or low mood when physical pain restricts daily activities or hobbies.
- Sensitivity to sympathy, where the individual may feel better with understanding and emotional support.

Psychological Symptoms: Ruta can address specific psychological responses that arise due to physical ailments:

• Anxiety about long-term recovery prospects, especially in athletes or physical occupations.

• Over concern with the body and physical health, particularly when movement is impaired.

• A tendency towards dwelling on the limitations imposed by injuries or strains.

Physical Symptoms: Ruta is particularly effective for a broad range of physical symptoms:

• Overuse Injuries: Ideal for treating conditions such as tennis elbow, golfer's elbow, and other repetitive strain injuries, where tendons and ligaments are overextended.

• Joint Pains: Effective in cases of arthritic pain or discomfort in the joints, especially if the pain feels as though the bone is bruised.

• Eye Strain: Beneficial for eye strain resulting from prolonged computer use, reading, or detailed work, often manifesting as a headache or a sensation of eye pressure.

• Sprains and Strains: Useful for sprains and strains that involve a feeling of bruising and stiffness, with pain that improves with gentle movement.

• Bone Bruises and Injuries: Assists in the healing of periosteal injuries or bruises, particularly following blows or impacts to bony areas.

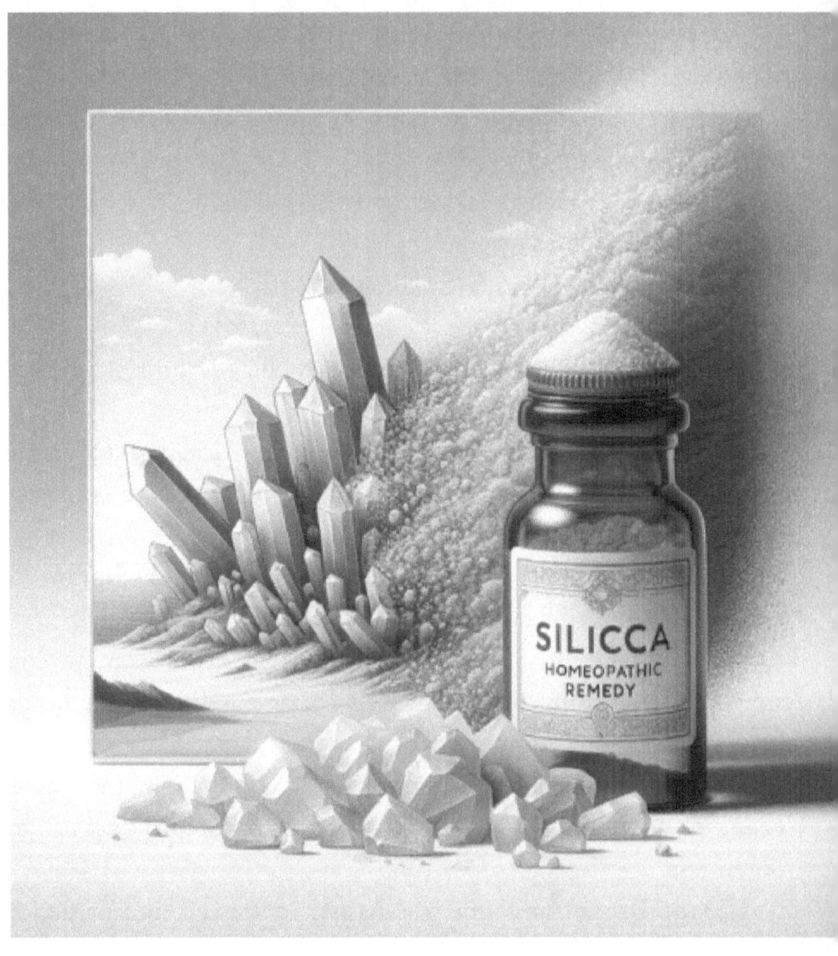
SILICCA
HOMEOPATHIC
REMEDY

Silica (Silicea):

Introduction: Silica, or Silicea, is a fundamental homeopathic remedy derived from silicon dioxide, a naturally occurring compound in quartz and human tissues. Esteemed in homeopathy for its profound ability to expel foreign bodies from the tissue and enhance the body's healing processes, Silica is particularly beneficial for conditions related to connective tissues, skin, and the nervous system. It is often indicated for individuals with a delicate constitution but a determined and strong-willed nature.

Homeopathic Preparation and Application: Adhering to homeopathic traditions, Silica is prepared through rigorous dilution and succussion, a process believed to imbue the substance with potent healing capabilities while mitigating potential adverse effects. This remedy is widely used to strengthen the constitution, promote the expulsion of splinters or foreign bodies, treat chronic infections, and support the healing of skin and connective tissue disorders.

Mental Symptoms: Silica is suited to individuals who display specific mental and cognitive characteristics:

• Lack of confidence and timidity, yet with a robust inner resolve and persistence.

• Mental fatigue, especially when faced with overwork or excessive intellectual demands.

• Anxious about small details, often leading to indecisiveness and procrastination.

Emotional Symptoms: The emotional profile of those benefiting from Silica includes:

• Sensitivity to criticism and a desire for approval, yet a strong sense of duty and responsibility.

• Tendency towards nervousness and anxiety, particularly regarding personal health or performance.

• Introversion and a preference for solitude despite a robust inner life and convictions.

Psychological Symptoms: Silica addresses various psychological aspects:

• Perseverance despite fear of failure, often pushing through challenges with quiet determination.

• Struggle with conflicting desires for independence and support from others.

• High standards for oneself and others, leading to disappointment when expectations are not met.

Physical Symptoms: Silica is particularly effective in treating a wide range of physical symptoms:

• Skin Conditions: Excellent for promoting the healing of acne, scars, and keloids and for conditions where the skin heals poorly or slowly.

• Connective Tissue Disorders: Aids treating weak connective tissues, including recurrent sprains and joint instability.

• Foreign Body Rejection: Facilitates the expulsion of splinters, glass shards, or other foreign bodies embedded in the skin.

• Chronic Infections: Useful in chronic infections where the body needs support to resolve the infection, such as recurrent tonsillitis or sinusitis.

• Nail and Hair Health: Strengthens brittle nails and hair, addressing issues like hair loss or split nails that are symptomatic of a more profound constitutional weakness.